Mastering the New Psychiatric Diagnoses

Three Practice Exams for Novices and Experts

Written by:
The 2013-2014 Psychiatry Residents and Fellows of Rutgers New Jersey Medical School

Edited by:
Samina S. Raja, MD
Petros Levounis, MD, MA

Newark, New Jersey
June 2014

ISBN-13: 9781497564640
ISBN-10: 1497564646
Library of Congress Control Number: 2014907382
CreateSpace Independent Publishing Platform
North Charleston, South Carolina

Preface

Welcome to "Mastering the New Psychiatric Diagnoses: Three Practice Exams for Novices and Experts"!

The book that you have in your hands is a labor of love, born out of the clinical experience, scholarship, hard work, and endless enthusiasm of the 30 doctors who served as the 2013-2014 residents and fellows of the Department of Psychiatry at Rutgers New Jersey Medical School.

For 14 weeks during the fall of 2013, 26 residents in Adult Psychiatry and 4 fellows in Child and Adolescent Psychiatry developed an innovative training method to study the new psychiatric diagnoses that came out of the Diagnostic and Statistical Manual, 5th Edition (DSM-5), of the American Psychiatric Association.

Each week, we studied a topic from the DSM-5 and generated a list of topics for further discussion. The following week, each resident was responsible for presenting a multiple choice question with explanation of the correct answer based on the previous week's topic. We critiqued the questions as a group and sent them back to their authors for further refinement. The 75 questions that make up the three exams of this volume are the result of this iterative group process, which turned out to be both highly educational and fun.

We hope this book will be helpful to medical students and psychiatry residents, as well as attending psychiatrists, counselors, nurses and nurse practitioners, psychologists, social workers, therapists, and other clinicians who are interested in mastering the new psychiatric diagnoses of the DSM-5.

Finally, we are deeply grateful to the faculty and staff of the Department of Psychiatry at Rutgers New Jersey Medical School for their encouragement, support, and patience as we kept revising the questions and answers of this volume.

Samina S. Raja, MD
Petros Levounis, MD, MA

Newark, New Jersey
June 2014

PSYCHIATRY RESIDENTS

PGY-4
Aikaterini Fineti, MD
Mahreen Raza, MD, Chief Resident
Nicole A. Guanci, MD, Chief Resident
Samina S. Raja, MD

PGY-3
Anbreen Khizar, MD
Atika Zubera, MD
Humaira Shoaib, MD
Noel M. Baker, MD
Shanel Chandra, MD
Shaojie Han, MD
Sonal Batra, MD
Susana Sanchez, MD
Tamkeen Khurshid, MD

PGY-2
Ankur S. Patel, MD
Meredith M. Brandon, MD
Michelle Benitez, MD
Noah D. Villegas, MD
Samina Y. Mirza, MD
Tshering W. Bhutia, MD
Wajid Hussain, MD

PGY-1
Afiah A. Ahsan, MD
Farha B. Motiwala, MD
Nahil S. Chohan, MD
Nayla Hariz, MD
Ritesh A. Amin, MD
Samir A. Qasim, MD

CHILD AND ADOLESCENT PSYCHIATRY FELLOWS

2nd Year
Cecilia Belardinelli, MD
Shirley Sostre-Oquendo, MD, JD

1st Year
Malgorzata Komza, MD
Riyad M. Rouf, MD

FACULTY

Barbara Fadem, PhD
Cheryl Kennedy, MD, Medical Student Clerkship Director
Diane Kaufman, MD
Douglas Opler, MD
Erin Zerbo, MD
Gerald Leventhal, PhD
Giovanni Caracci, MD
Gregorio Castillo, MD
Jacob Lindenthal, PhD
Jocelynda Udasco, MD
Lily Arora, MD
Mukti Chakrabarti, MD
Nadia Mirza, MD
Najeeb Hussain, MD, Residency Training Director
Paula Pesci, MD
Petros Levounis, MD, MA, Chair
Rashi Aggarwal, MD, Associate Residency Training
    Director
Sabina Mushtaq, MD
Steven Schleifer, MD
Stuart Belenker, MD
Tolga Taneli, MD, Child and Adolescent Psychiatry
    Fellowship Director
Ye-Ming (Jimmy) Sun, MD

ADMINISTRATIVE STAFF

Carmen Torres
Dorothy Lemon
Ed Warhola, Department Administrator
Ileana Hernandez
Jacqueline Rivas
Rajashri Patel
Sheila Morris

Table of Contents

Part I

The Three Exams

Test #1

-1-
What is the most common comorbidity in bipolar disorder?

A. Attention-Deficit/Hyperactivity Disorder
B. Substance Use Disorder
C. Anxiety Disorder
D. Impulse-Control Disorder
E. Eating Disorder

-2-
Which of the following is the most common eating disorder that can co-occur in bipolar II disorder?

A. Pica
B. Binge-Eating Disorder
C. Anorexia Nervosa
D. Bulimia Nervosa
E. Rumination Disorder

-3-

What is the estimated lifetime risk of suicide in individuals with bipolar disorder as compared to the general population?

A. 50 times
B. 35 times
C. 15 times
D. 5 times
E. 1.5 times

-4-

A 20-year-old college sophomore presents to her school's counseling center. She reports her parents are concerned about her rapid rate of speech and told her she is becoming "manic" like her uncle Charlie who has a gambling problem. She reports otherwise feeling "great" and only came today because her parents threatened to take back her credit card unless she complied with today's visit. She reports maintaining good grades, has lots of energy, and can function well despite only 3 hours of sleep per night. She reports finishing her homework so quickly that she has time to focus on new projects, including re-painting the walls in her room. She adds that everything was going well until she started to buy some extra clothes online with her parent's credit card and her parents forced her to return the items. The presence of which of the following would help distinguish between bipolar I and bipolar II disorder?

A. Patient's symptoms have lasted 7 days
B. Patient's friends notice a change in behavior from baseline
C. Patient doesn't feel anything is wrong with her
D. Patient is paranoid about others stealing her brilliant ideas
E. Patient's uncle has a history of bipolar I disorder

-5-

A 19-year-old college student is brought to the psychiatrist by her mother for being 'moody' for the last 3 years. According to the mother, the patient can alternate between being happy and sad. For a few days she is cheerful, spending time with friends and family, and staying up 2-3 nights in a row to prepare for exams and assignments that are not due for weeks. This is followed by several days of irritable mood, isolating in her room, not talking to family, and sleeping all day long. Her mother further states that there are only a few weeks in between when she is either not too irritable or overly pleasant and nice. The mother read on the Internet about mood disorders and became concerned about her daughter's mental health. The patient responded by saying "My mom is overly concerned, I am fine what else would you expect from a 20-year- old?!" Medical illness and drug abuse have been ruled out. What is the most likely diagnosis?

A. Unspecified mood and related disorder
B. Bipolar II disorder
C. Cyclothymic disorder
D. Bipolar and related disorder with atypical features
E. Cluster B personality disorder

-6-
Which of the following is NOT consistent with a diagnosis of disruptive mood dysregulation disorder?

A. Severe, recurrent temper outbursts manifested verbally and/or behaviorally out of proportion to the provocation
B. The temper outbursts are appropriate for the patient's developmental level
C. Outbursts occur 3 or more times per week
D. Outbursts occur for at least 12 months
E. The diagnosis cannot be made before age 6 or after age 18

-7-
In distinguishing grief from a major depressive disorder, it is useful to consider that in grief the predominant affect is:

A. Persistently depressed mood and inability to anticipate happiness and pleasure
B. Feelings of emptiness and loss
C. Severe recurrent temper outbursts with irritable mood
D. Elated mood with grandiose delusions
E. Self-critical or pessimistic ruminations

-8-

Approximately what percentage of women will experience the onset of a major depressive episode during pregnancy or postpartum period?

A. 5%
B. 15%
C. 30%
D. 50%
E. 75%

-9-

Compared to individuals with major depressive disorder, those with persistent depressive disorder (dysthymia) are at higher risk for which of the following comorbidities?

A. Bipolar disorder
B. Schizophrenia
C. Substance use disorders
D. Cluster A personality disorders
E. Posttraumatic stress disorder

-10-

A 50-year-old man presents to outpatient clinic this morning complaining of mildly depressed mood. He has been irritable, fatigued, experiencing headaches, temper outbursts, and having difficulty concentrating. He has never felt down before and lately has been exercising and eating healthier. Just yesterday he decided to eliminate sweets from his diet and give up caffeinated beverages, as he is a daily soda and coffee drinker. He drinks alcohol socially and his last alcoholic beverage was 3 nights ago. Which of the following explains his presenting symptoms?

A. Disruptive mood dysregulation disorder
B. Substance-Induced Depressive Disorder
C. Unspecified Depressive Disorder
D. Caffeine Withdrawal
E. Alcohol Withdrawal

-11-

Which of the following is the only non-substance-related addictive disorder recognized in the DSM-5 chapter on addictive disorders?

A. Gambling disorder
B. Internet gaming disorder
C. Social media addictive disorder
D. Compulsive computer gaming
E. Compulsive shopping

-12-
Which of the following symptoms develop within several hours to a few days after cessation of alcohol to indicate alcohol withdrawal?

A. Nystagmus and incoordination
B. Dysphoric mood and rhinorrhea
C. Headache and flu-like symptoms
D. Irritability and decreased appetite
E. Insomnia and nausea/vomiting

-13-
A 21-year-old Caucasian man was recently diagnosed with paranoid schizophrenia. After a few doses of an atypical antipsychotic, he wakes up one morning confused, pale, and dysarthric. He is rigid throughout his extremities and warm to touch. His parents rush him to the ED for medical attention. Vital signs include: temperature 101°F, blood pressure 145/85, heart rate 112, and respiratory rate 22. Neuroleptic malignant syndrome (NMS) is highly suspected. Preliminary workup reveals leukocytosis, elevated creatine kinase and liver enzymes, and normal CT findings, consistent with NMS. Which of the following is also associated with this syndrome?

A. Metabolic alkalosis
B. Increased serum iron concentration
C. Generalized slowing on electroencephalography (EEG)
D. Agranulocytosis
E. Increased opening pressure on spinal tap

-14-

A 72-year-old man with a history of hypertension and hyper-cholesterolemia presents to your clinic with his wife for an evaluation of memory problems. According to his wife, in the past few years after his stroke, he has become more forgetful of dates and family members' names. He gets confused more easily, often forgetting what he is doing and where he is going, leading to him wandering outside the house and being unable to drive. He also is unable to pay the bills anymore. Lately, after a hospitalization for a "mini stroke," he has been having difficulty speaking, described as "forgetting what things are called" and is having difficulty dressing and feeding himself. Which of the following is the most likely diagnosis?

A. Major Cognitive Disorder due to Alzheimer's Disease
B. Major Frontotemporal Neurocognitive Disorder
C. Major Vascular Neurocognitive Disorder
D. Major Neurocognitive Disorder with Lewy Bodies
E. Delirium

-15-

A 70-year-old woman with a history of alcohol use disorder is day 10 of hospital admission from her assisted living facility for dehydration due to acute gallstone pancreatitis and protracted vomiting. After endoscopic removal of the gallstone in the common bile duct, she beings to improve and remains on parenteral intake due to continued vomiting and nausea. She remained in the hospital for vomiting but after it resolved she developed acute inattention and confusion 3 days ago. She is slightly better during the morning. On exam she is able to tell you her name but is disoriented to time and place. She has difficulty looking to the left and appears to be picking at something on her clothing. The rest of the exam is unremarkable. Her CT scan is negative for acute changes, including hemorrhage. Routine labs are normal as are amylase, lipase, lactate, and bilirubin levels. She is not able to focus to complete a MMSE. What is the most likely diagnosis?

A. Major Neurocognitive Disorder Due to Alzheimer's Disease
B. Major Vascular Neurocognitive Disorder
C. Alcohol withdrawal delirium
D. Delirium due to vitamin deficiency
E. None of the above

-16-

Which one of the following neurocognitive disorders includes visual hallucinations and parkinsonism?

A. Neurocognitive disorder due to Prion disease
B. Neurocognitive disorder due to Huntington's disease
C. Neurocognitive disorder due to HIV infection
D. Neurocognitive disorder with Lewy Bodies
E. Frontotemporal neurocognitive disorder

-17-

A 48-year-old former football player, now private football coach, presents to your office accompanied by his wife. He reports coming to your office on his wife's insistence due concerns of his gradual decline in concentration over the past 3 years. He continues to work and remains independent. There are no personality changes noted by his wife. Family history is insignificant. There is no known history of traumatic brain injury. Medical workup performed 6 months ago, including bloodwork, chest x-ray, and CT head did not show any findings of significance to explain his symptoms. He scores a perfect 30 out of 30 on the MMSE performed in your office. He is referred for neuropsychiatric testing and the results come back showing that he is between 1-2 standard deviations below the mean in tests of complex attention while other areas of testing do not show any significant abnormalities. What is the most likely diagnosis?

A. Mild neurocognitive disorder due to Alzheimer's disease
B. Mild neurocognitive disorder
C. Major neurocognitive disorder
D. Mild neurocognitive disorder due to traumatic brain injury
E. Major neurocognitive disorder due to traumatic brain injury

-18-

Which of the following helps differentiate major neuro-cognitive disorder from mild neurocognitive disorder?

A. Concern of the individual
B. Impairment documented by neuropsychological testing
C. Interference with independence in everyday activities
D. Comorbid delirium
E. Comorbid psychiatric disorder

-19-

Which of the following is one of the six cognitive domains used to define the various neurocognitive disorders?

A. Language
B. Social cognition
C. Abstraction
D. Both A & B
E. Both A & C

-20-
A 38-year-old meat factory worker is admitted to inpatient psychiatry for bizarre behavior. Neurology was consulted for newly developed ataxia and myoclonus. The patient becomes mute with major neurocognitive decline within days and is transferred to the neurology service. A few days later she dies in the intensive care unit. The patient was single with no children and did not have any major medical problems. What is the most likely diagnosis?

A. Major neurocognitive disorder due to prion disease
B. Major neurocognitive disorder due to HIV infection
C. Major neurocognitive disorder due to Parkinson's disease
D. Major neurocognitive disorder with Lewy bodies
E. Major neurocognitive disorder due to Huntington's disease

-21-
A 70-year-old Caucasian man with no prior psychiatric history is admitted to the hospital for congestive heart failure and found to have severe aortic stenosis. Per nursing staff, he has been getting agitated, pulling out intravenous lines, and demanding to leave the hospital to walk his dogs. On evaluation, he is pleasantly smiling and appears to be in no acute painful or emotional distress. He is aware he is in the hospital, but thinks the year is 1956. Which of the following is a feature of delirium that can help differentiate it from dementia?

A. Memory loss
B. Inattention
C. Fluctuating course
D. Disorganized thinking
E. Agitation

-22-

A 45-year-old woman presents to the emergency room with complaints of increased urinary frequency, headaches, backaches, lower abdominal pain, and numbness in her fingers for the past seven months. She reports that she has been missing deadlines at work due to appointments with different doctors and constantly worries about her health. She was informed by her doctor that all her basic labs, including abdominal ultrasound are within normal limits. What is the correct diagnosis?

A. Illness anxiety disorder
B. Somatic symptom disorder
C. Factitious disorder
D. Brief somatic symptom disorder
E. Malingering

-23-
A 26-year-old non-combat Iraqi War army veteran presents complaining of six month history of anxiety. He reports intense anxiety of being outside his home alone or in large crowds of people. He fears that escape in such situations may be difficult or that he will not be able to get help if he develops panic-like symptoms, such as palpitations or dizziness, which he experienced once before during a Fourth of July parade. He recognizes that his anxiety is excessive and he feels sad, because it has limited his social life. When asked about his military experiences, he mentions he witnessed several dead bodies in Afghanistan but does not endorse any re-experiencing symptoms, such as nightmares or flashbacks. He states he has moved on from his military experience and the discipline he gained while in active duty has helped him do well in his civilian IT job. He has a supportive wife and two young healthy children, ages three and five at home. He is a life-time nonsmoker, drinks rarely at social occasions, and denies illicit drug use now or ever in the past. What is his diagnosis?

A. Posttraumatic stress disorder (PTSD)
B. Panic disorder
C. Agoraphobia
D. Unspecified anxiety disorder
E. Separation anxiety disorder

-24-
The criteria for posttraumatic stress disorder have changed in DSM-5. The previous three clusters were: re-experiencing, avoidance, and hyperarousal symptoms. In DSM-5, the avoidance/numbing cluster has been divided into two distinct categories: persistent avoidance and which of the following?

A. Problems with concentration
B. Sleep disturbance
C. Distressing dreams
D. Negative alterations in cognitions and mood
E. Hypervigilance

-25-
A 24-year-old student presents to outpatient clinic complaining of intense "anxiety attacks," characterized by feeling extremely nervous and shaky, with sweaty palms. These symptoms occur when he is meeting new people for the first time, asking questions in class, or making oral presentations. Symptoms last until he is alone or in the company of close friends or family members. Symptoms occur when he has to talk in front of others and he is constantly worried about being embarrassed. Due to these symptoms for the past year, he avoids participating in class and going to parties with too many new faces. Which of the following is the most likely diagnosis?

A. Panic disorder with agoraphobia
B. Social anxiety disorder
C. Generalized anxiety disorder
D. Panic disorder without agoraphobia
E. Adjustment disorder

Test #2

-26-
A mother brings her 8-year-old son for evaluation. She explains for the past six months her child has been irritable, throwing tantrums, and seems to "freeze" while awaiting for the school bus, and "clings" to her when it arrives. She now finds herself driving him to and from school, as he has similar reactions while waiting for the bus to return home. The mother reports at home the child is comfortable and does not display any anxiety symptoms. Which of the following is the most likely diagnosis?

A. Separation Anxiety disorder
B. Specific phobia, situational type
C. Agoraphobia
D. Panic disorder
E. Panic attack

-27-

A 17-year-old high school student has been engaging in nightly binge-eating episodes for the past 4 months. She eats large quantities of fast food, such as 12 pieces of fried chicken, 3 orders of mashed potatoes, and 2 slices of pie in a 2 hour period while alone in her bedroom. Afterwards, she feels full and disgusted with herself. During the day, she watches her calories and has an adequate intake of food, but also uses laxatives and purges in the school bathroom. She constantly checks herself in the mirror to make sure she doesn't look fat. She wants to be thin and beautiful like the models she sees in fashion magazines. Her friends constantly reassure her that she looks fine—in fact, they tell her she is too thin. Her BMI is 15. What personality disorder is most closely associated with her eating disorder?

A. Borderline personality disorder
B. Obsessive compulsive personality disorder
C. Histrionic personality disorder
D. Narcissistic personality disorder
E. Avoidant personality disorder

-28-
A 27-year-old respiratory therapist with no prior psychia-try history is admitted to the medical floor with intractable vomiting for the third time within the past six months. About a year prior to the onset of vomiting episodes, the patient was briefly hospitalized after a motor vehicle accident. The cause of vomiting has not been identified despite extensive diagnostic testing. The patient insists that there should be a medical reason behind her vomiting. Per nursing staff, the patient vomits much less than she reports. No evidence of external secondary gain to explain the patient's behavior can be identified. What is the most likely diagnosis?

A. Somatic symptom disorder
B. Malingering
C. Conversion disorder
D. Factitious disorder
E. Delusional disorder

-29-

An 18-year-old woman is brought in by her mother because she has witnessed her eating toilet paper. The mother also reports her daughter has been vomiting frequently. On physical exam you observe a tall thin woman with a BMI of 17 kg/m², with no apparent physical abnormalities. On interview she eventually admits to consuming both tissues and toilet paper because they have no calories. She also admits she sometimes eats large amounts of food and then uses laxatives or purges to compensate for her behavior because she feels fat. What is the most likely diagnosis?

A. Pica
B. Anorexia nervosa
C. Binge eating disorder
D. Bulimia nervosa
E. Avoidant/restrictive food intake disorder

-30-

Which of the following criteria best differentiates bulimia nervosa from binge-eating disorder?

A. Sense of lack of control
B. Feelings of shame or guilt
C. Normal body weight
D. Recurrent inappropriate compensatory behavior
E. Frequent attempts at dieting

-31-
Which of the following is a key feature of factitious disorder?

A. Somatic symptoms
B. Misrepresentation of signs and symptoms
C. External gain associated with illness
D. Absence of another medical disorder that may cause the symptoms
E. Normal physical exam and laboratory tests

-32-
Which of the following is correct regarding the diagnosis of intermittent explosive disorder?

A. Aggressive outbursts must be physical in nature
B. Aggressive outbursts can be either physical or verbal in nature
C. Chronological age is at least 9 years
D. Destruction of property or physical injury must occur
E. Outbursts are committed to achieve a tangible objective, such as money, power, or intimidation

-33-
A 52-year-old man eats at Old Country Buffet once a week. He eats more at the table than anyone else around him and seems to lack a sense of control over his excessive eating. He feels he deserves to eat what he wants after working long days on the farm. Despite his increasing girth, he feels his overeating is not problematic. His primary care physician educates him about the consequences of being overweight. He tells the doctor "I'll think about it" and appears to mean it. He decides to exercise 30 minutes on the weekends to lose weight. What is his most likely diagnosis?

A. Bulimia nervosa
B. Binge-eating disorder
C. Anorexia nervosa, binge-eating type
D. No DSM-5 diagnosis
E. Other specified feeding or eating disorder

-34-
A 30-year-old woman comes to clinic complaining of recurrent episodes of visual distortions, hypoemotionality, feeling robotic, and detached from her whole self. She is fearful of going crazy and having irreversible brain damage due to her symptoms. Which of the following is true about the disorder this woman most likely has?

A. Reality testing remains intact
B. There is high comorbidity with posttraumatic stress disorder
C. It commonly co-occurs with schizotypal personality disorder
D. It commonly occurs in women
E. It is usually caused by hallucinogens

-35-

A 22-year-old woman comes to your office complaining of multiple scab marks on her upper extremities and an unrelenting urge to pick her skin. She reports she feels less tense after picking her skin, and upon further interview it appears the skin picking is not in response to an obsession or done to prevent something bad from happening to her. She denies visual or tactile hallucinations, does not believe she has a rash or infection, and does not feel her arms are otherwise deformed. She denies alcohol or illicit drug use and has no medical problems. Due to her scabs, she has to take off from work and avoids going out socially. Which of the following is the most likely diagnosis?

A. Body dysmorphic disorder
B. Excoriation disorder
C. Obsessive compulsive disorder
D. Adjustment disorder
E. Generalized anxiety disorder

-36-

A couple recently adopted a 4-year-old child from an orphanage in a war-stricken country. Very little is known about the child's history, except that she lost all her family at 2 months of age. She was found barely breathing in the rubble of a destroyed neighborhood. She was brought to a hospital, then to several shelters, and finally taken up by an orphanage in a small village quite far from where she was originally found. The adoptive parents are noticing that the child barely talks, has poor eye contact, appears sad and fearful for no reason, and has frequent unexplained episodes of irritability. She interacts poorly with the parents and other children. What is the most likely diagnosis?

A. Autism spectrum disorder
B. Intellectual developmental disorder
C. Major depressive episode
D. Reactive attachment disorder
E. Normal reaction to extreme stressors

-37-

Personality disorders should not be diagnosed on the basis of problems associated with:

A. Interpersonal functioning
B. Affectivity
C. Cognition
D. Impulse Control
E. Acculturation following immigration

-38-
A 21-year-old man presents to his primary medical doctor with his mother for an annual check-up. She reports wanting a second opinion for his "weird behavior." She reports that the patient has always been eccentric. She reports that he believes he has extra-sensory perception (ESP) and speaks as if he were a fortune-teller to family members. He has also has a tendency to wear odd combinations of patterns and has not made any friends while away at college. He has never complained of mood symptoms or auditory or visual hallucinations. Which of the following is the most likely diagnosis?

A. Schizophrenia
B. Schizophreniform Disorder
C. Schizoaffective Disorder
D. Schizotypal Personality Disorder
E. Schizoid Personality Disorder

-39-
Which of the following personality disorders is part of the schizophrenia spectrum of disorders?

A. Paranoid personality disorder
B. Schizoid personality disorder
C. Schizotypal personality disorder
D. Dependent personality disorder
E. Avoidant personality disorder

-40-

Why were subtypes of schizophrenia (i.e., paranoid, disorganized, catatonic, undifferentiated, residual) removed from the DSM-5?

A. Poor validity
B. Low reliability
C. Limited diagnostic stability
D. A & B
E. All of the above

-41-

Which of the following is true concerning individuals diagnosed with attention-deficit/hyperactivity disorder?

A. Symptoms must cause impairment prior to age 7
B. Inattentive or hyperactive-impulsive symptoms were present prior to age 12
C. There is no age requirement for onset of symptoms as long as there is impairment at home and school
D. Inattentive symptoms occur more commonly in males
E. None of the above is true.

-42-
Which of the following is true regarding Tourette's Disorder?

A. The onset of symptoms must occur prior to age 12
B. Motor and vocal tics occur simultaneously
C. Tics must persist for at least 2 years
D. Both motor and vocal tics must occur at some time during the illness
E. Either motor or vocal tics must occur during the illness

-43-
Childhood-onset fluency disorder involves problems with:

A. Sound and syllable repetitions
B. Social uses of verbal and nonverbal communication
C. Social-emotional reciprocity
D. Reduced vocabulary, including both word knowledge and use
E. Impaired ability to use vocabulary and explain a series of events

-44-
Which of the following describes a condition or disorder which would be properly diagnosed as "Other Specified Sexual Dysfunction"?

A. Medical-induced sexual dysfunction
B. Sexual aversion
C. Erectile dysfunction
D. Female sexual interest/arousal disorder
E. Delayed ejaculation

-45-
Which of the following is classified as an anxiety disorder?

A. Specific phobia
B. Obsessive-compulsive disorder
C. Selective mutism
D. Both A & B
E. Both A & C

-46-
The diagnosis of autism spectrum disorder includes all of the following, EXCEPT?

A. Deficits in social communication
B. Deficits in social interaction
C. Deficits in developing and maintaining relationships
D. Sound and syllable repetitions
E. Deficits in non-verbal communication behaviors

-47-
For a diagnosis of hypersomnolence disorder, which of the following is true?

A. The hypersomnolence occurs at least two times per week, for at least two months
B. The hypersomnolence occurs at least five times per week, for at least one month
C. The hypersomnolence occurs at least three times per week, for at least three months
D. The hypersomnolence occurs for at least six months
E. The hypersomnolence occurs for at least one year

-48-
A 10-year-old girl with no past psychiatric history is brought for mental health evaluation after her mother noticed a change in her behavior for the past 7-8 months. The mother explains that the patient often loses her temper, has been vindictive at times, and recently confronted her school principal after she was suspended. Which of the following is the most accurate diagnosis?

A. Intermittent explosive disorder
B. Conduct disorder
C. Oppositional defiant disorder
D. Antisocial personality disorder
E. Borderline personality disorder

-49-
A 35-year-old man presents complaining of very poor sexual desire. He states that he has been having decreased interest in romantic relationships and sexual activity for over a year. He reports barely thinking about sex and not having the fantasies he used to have. Though he has never been much of a sexual creature he finds his nearly absent sexual desire problematic. He reports that he has been in a few relationships in the past and is currently single. He has stable employment, owns his house, and reports no medical problems. He does not smoke, drink or use any illicit drugs, and states that he is content professionally. What is the most likely diagnosis?

A. Major depressive disorder
B. Gender dysphoria
C. Unspecified sexual dysfunction
D. Male hypoactive sexual desire disorder
E. No psychiatric disorder

-50-
An 18-year-old man with no significant medical history presents to his primary care physician with complaints of excessive tiredness and daytime napping for the past 6 months. He is currently a freshman in college and is experiencing difficulty staying awake, especially during class. He notes that approximately 5-6 times per week he suddenly "collapses," associated at times with significant bruising. His BMI is 22 and routine labs reveal no abnormalities. Which of the following would the most appropriate next test to perform?

A. Magnetic resonance imaging of the brain
B. Lumbar puncture with cerebrospinal fluid analysis
C. Nerve conduction studies
D. Electroencephalogram
E. Urine toxicology

Test #3

-51-
A 28-year-old man with history of schizoaffective disorder presents to the emergency department after police find him agitated on the streets. He receives haloperidol 5mg intramuscularly 4 times in the course of 24 hours and is admitted to the inpatient psychiatric service. On day 2 of hospitalization he develops a painful twisting of his neck. Vital signs and laboratory tests are within normal limits. Which of the following is the most likely cause?

A. Medication-induced acute dystonia
B. Medication-induced akathisia
C. Tardive dyskinesia
D. Neuroleptic malignant syndrome
E. Medication-induced Parkinsonism

-52-

Which of the following is NOT considered to be one of the symptoms of caffeine intoxication?

A. Restlessness
B. Flushed Face
C. Rambling flow of speech
D. Periods of inexhaustibility
E. Headache

-53-

A 17-year-old teenager is brought to the emergency department by his family. They report he is aggressive, confused, and producing nonsensical speech. His skin appears erythematous and dry; his pupils are dilated and he is noted to have involuntary eye movements. The family reports the patient had just returned from a party prior to presenting with above symptoms. What is the most likely diagnosis?

A. Cannabis intoxication
B. PCP intoxication
C. Alcohol intoxication
D. Caffeine withdrawal
E. Cocaine intoxication

-54-
A 19-year-old patient is brought to the emergency department by EMS for assaultive behavior. The patient states that he is "just fine," but refuses to change into a gown and is cursing and yelling at staff. He finally agrees to change and is examined by the resident psychiatrist. He is noted on mental status examination to have psychomotor retardation, slurred speech, and impaired judgment. Eye examination reveals nystagmus. Other positive findings include depressed reflexes and unsteady gait. The patient is most likely intoxication with which of the following?

A. PCP
B. Inhalant
C. Cocaine
D. Opioid
E. Cannabis

-55-
Which of the following is true when differentiating mild or major neurocognitive disorder (NCD) with Lewy bodies from NCD due to Parkinson's disease?

A. In Parkinson's disease, cognitive decline occurs in the context of established Parkinson's disease; in NCD with Lewy bodies, cognitive symptoms occur before or concurrently with spontaneous parkinsonism
B. In Parkinson's disease, cognitive decline occurs before motor symptoms associated with Parkinson's disease; in NCD with Lewy bodies, cognitive symptoms occur after motor symptoms
C. Patients with Parkinson's disease are more likely to report visual hallucinations
D. NCD with Lewy bodies occurs more frequently in females
E. Parkinson's disease is a synucleinopathy due to alpha-synuclein misfolding and aggregation

-56-
Which trinucleotide repeat is observed in the gene that encodes the huntingtin protein in Huntington's disease?

A. CAT
B. CAG
C. CAC
D. TAG
E. CCG

-57-
Loss of consciousness in mild traumatic brain injury (TBI) typically lasts for how long?

A. Less than 15 minutes
B. Less than 30 minutes
C. 30 minutes to 24 hours
D. Greater than 24 hours
E. Greater than 36 hours

-58-
What is the most common cause of a traumatic brain injury (TBI)?

A. Falls
B. Motor vehicle accident
C. Sports concussions
D. Combat-related blasts
E. Gunshot wound

-59-
An example of an assessment for sustained attention is:

A. Measuring time taken to put together a design of blocks
B. Hearing numbers and letters read and asking to count only numbers
C. Pressing a button every time a bell is heard
D. Rapidly tapping one's feet while carrying a conversation
E. Shifting from ordering objects by color to ordering by size

-60-

Major risk factors for mild or major vascular neurocognitive (NCD) disorder include:

A. History of repeated falls
B. Thyroid dysfunction
C. Smoking
D. Low homocysteine levels
E. Sleep disorder

-61-

Which of the following DOES NOT occur in delusional disorder?

A. More than one delusion
B. Bizarre delusions
C. Impaired functioning
D. Hallucinations
E. Brief major depressive episodes

-62-

Obsessive-compulsive disorder (OCD) is characterized by:

A. Intrusive thoughts and repetitive behaviors
B. Either intrusive thoughts or repetitive behaviors
C. Excessive worrying
D. Guilty ruminations
E. Recurrent, pleasurable thoughts

-63-

Recurrent and intense sexual arousal from observing an unsuspecting person who is naked, in the process of disrobing, or engaging in sexual activity is:

A. Voyeuristic disorder
B. Exhibitionistic disorder
C. Frotteuristic disorder
D. Sexual sadism disorder
E. Fetishtic disorder

-64-

What is the minimum length of time symptoms should be present for a diagnosis of delayed ejaculation?

A. 2 weeks
B. 6 weeks
C. 1-3 months
D. 6 months
E. 12 months

-65-

Alexithymia, a common occurrence in men diagnosed with psychogenic erectile dysfunction, is defined as:

A. Persistently low mood
B. Anxious affect
C. Intense emotional reactions
D. Affective blunting
E. Deficits in cognitive processing of emotions

-66-
Taiijin kyofusho is:

A. "Interpersonal fear disorder"
B. "Fright"
C. "Weakness of the nervous system"
D. "Thinking too much"
E. "Wind attacks"

-67-
How are illness anxiety disorder and somatic symptom disorder similar?

A. High levels of anxiety about health are experienced
B. Significant somatic symptoms are present
C. The individual performs excessive health-related behaviors
D. A & B
E. A & C

-68-
Disorders most commonly comorbid with pica are:

A. Autism spectrum disorder
B. Intellectual disability
C. Obsessive-compulsive disorder
D. A & B
E. A & C

-69-

Rumination disorder is:

A. Repeated regurgitation of food; the food is either re-chewed, re-swallowed, or spit out
B. Excessive attention to one's own distress in the setting of depressive symptoms
C. Characterized by recurrent, unwanted intrusive thoughts
D. Characterized by excessive time spent before making decisions commonly in the setting of a perfectionistic personality style
E. Related to excessive anxiety over making decisions related to everyday matters

-70-

Avoidant/restrictive food intake disorder is:

A. Avoidance of food based on the sensory characteristics of food
B. Avoidance of eating food in social situations secondary to anxiety about embarrassing oneself in public
C. Can be related to dependence on enteral feeding or oral nutritional supplements
D. A & B
E. A & C

-71-
Which of the following is true about dissociative amnesia?

A. Non-epileptic seizures may accompany dissociative amnesia
B. Is irreversible because neurobiological damage prevents memory storage and retrieval
C. Individuals with dissociative amnesia are frequently unaware of their memory problems
D. A & B
E. A & C

-72-
Encopresis is:

A. Repeated voiding of urine into bed or clothes
B. Not diagnosed until a child has reached a chronological of at least 6 years
C. More common in females
D. Often comorbid with urinary tract infections
E. Most often intentional

-73-
What is the core feature of gender dysphoria?

A. Marked incongruence between one's experienced/
   expressed gender and assigned gender
B. A strong preference for playmates of the other gender
C. A strong dislike of one's sexual anatomy
D. A strong preference for cross-gender roles
E. A strong desire for the sexual characteristics that
   match one's experienced gender

-74-
The prevalence of which of the following is higher in children with enuresis than in children without enuresis:

A. Autism spectrum disorder
B. Behavioral symptoms
C. Anxiety disorders
D. Tourette's disorder
E. Attention-deficit/hyperactivity disorders

-75-
Which of the following is an example of a phase of life
problem?

A. Bullying or intimidation by another individual
B. Retiring
C. Getting married
D. B & C
E. All of the above

Part II

The Three Exams with Answers and Explanations

Test #1

-1-
What is the most common comorbidity in bipolar disorder?

A. Attention-Deficit/Hyperactivity Disorder
B. Substance Use Disorder
C. Anxiety Disorder
D. Impulse-Control Disorder
E. Eating Disorder

Answer C: Anxiety disorders, such as panic attacks, social phobia, or a specific phobia, occur in approximately 75% of individuals with bipolar disorder. The other answer choices occur in over half of individuals with bipolar I disorder. *Note*: Adults with bipolar disorder also have higher rates of co-occurring medical conditions. Metabolic syndrome and migraines are more common in individuals with bipolar disorder than in the general population.

-2-

Which of the following is the most common eating disorder that can co-occur in bipolar II disorder?

A. Pica
B. Binge-Eating Disorder
C. Anorexia Nervosa
D. Bulimia Nervosa
E. Rumination Disorder

Answer B: Approximately 14% of individuals with bipolar II disorder have at least one lifetime eating disorder, with binge-eating disorder being the most common. When present, eating disorders are associated strongly with mood states and are more prominent in depressive episodes than in mania. Autism spectrum disorders, and to a lesser degree, schizophrenia can be comorbid with pica.

-3-

What is the estimated lifetime risk of suicide in individuals with bipolar disorder as compared to the general population?

A. 50 times
B. 35 times
C. 15 times
D. 5 times
E. 1.5 times

Answer C: The lifetime risk of suicide in patients with bipolar disorder is estimated to be at least 15 times that of general population.

-4-

A 20-year-old college sophomore presents to her school's counseling center. She reports her parents are concerned about her rapid rate of speech and told her she is becoming "manic" like her uncle Charlie who has a gambling problem. She reports otherwise feeling "great" and only came today because her parents threatened to take back her credit card unless she complied with today's visit. She reports maintaining good grades, has lots of energy, and can function well despite only 3 hours of sleep per night. She reports finishing her homework so quickly that she has time to focus on new projects, including re-painting the walls in her room. She adds that everything was going well until she started to buy some extra clothes online with her parent's credit card and her parents forced her to return the items. The presence of which of the following would help distinguish between bipolar I and bipolar II disorder?

A. Patient's symptoms have lasted 7 days
B. Patient's friends notice a change in behavior from baseline
C. Patient doesn't feel anything is wrong with her
D. **Patient is paranoid about others stealing her brilliant ideas**
E. Patient's uncle has a history of bipolar I disorder

Answer D: No psychosis is present in bipolar II disorder. All other choices can be present in both bipolar I or II.

-5-

A 19-year-old college student is brought to the psychiatrist by her mother for being 'moody' for the last 3 years. According to the mother, the patient can alternate between being happy and sad. For a few days she is cheerful, spending time with friends and family, and staying up 2-3 nights in a row to prepare for exams and assignments that are not due for weeks. This is followed by several days of irritable mood, isolating in her room, not talking to family, and sleeping all day long. Her mother further states that there are only a few weeks in between when she is either not too irritable or overly pleasant and nice. The mother read on the Internet about mood disorders and became concerned about her daughter's mental health. The patient responded by saying "My mom is overly concerned, I am fine what else would you expect from a 20-year- old?!" Medical illness and drug abuse have been ruled out. What is the most likely diagnosis?

A. Unspecified mood and related disorder
B. Bipolar II disorder
C. Cyclothymic disorder
D. Bipolar and related disorder with atypical features
E. Cluster B personality disorder

Answer C: In cyclothymic disorder, there are numerous periods of hypomanic symptoms that do not meet the criteria for hypomanic episode and there are numerous periods with depressive symptoms that do not meet the criteria of major depressive episodes. The individual should not be without the symptoms for more than 2 months at a time.

-6-

Which of the following is NOT consistent with a diagnosis of disruptive mood dysregulation disorder?

A. Severe, recurrent temper outbursts manifested verbally and/or behaviorally out of proportion to the provocation
B. The temper outbursts are appropriate for the patient's developmental level
C. Outbursts occur 3 or more times per week
D. Outbursts occur for at least 12 months
E. The diagnosis cannot be made before age 6 or after age 18

Answer B: Disruptive mood dysregulation disorder consists of temper tantrums that occur at least 3 times per week over at least a 12 month period. These outbursts occur out of proportion to the stimulus. The diagnosis cannot be made before age 6 or after age 18. The temper tantrums are NOT appropriate for the patient's developmental level.

-7-

In distinguishing grief from a major depressive disorder, it is useful to consider that in grief the predominant affect is:

A. Persistently depressed mood and inability to antici-pate happiness and pleasure
B. Feelings of emptiness and loss
C. Severe recurrent temper outbursts with irritable mood
D. Elated mood with grandiose delusions
E. Self-critical or pessimistic ruminations

Answer B: Grief is accompanied by feelings of emptiness and loss. The dysphoria is likely to decrease in intensity over days to weeks and occurs in waves. The pain in grief may be accompanied by positive emotions and humor. The thought content in grief involves a preoccupation with thoughts and memories of the deceased. Also, in grief self-esteem is preserved. In contrast, a major depressive episode is characterized by a persistently depressed mood, self-criticism, feelings of worthlessness, and an inability to anticipate happiness or pleasure.

-8-

Approximately what percentage of women will experience the onset of a major depressive episode during pregnancy or postpartum period?

A. 5%
B. 15%
C. 30%
D. 50%
E. 75%

Answer A: Mood episodes can have their onset either during pregnancy or postpartum. Approximately 3-6% of women will experience the onset of a major depressive episode during pregnancy or in the weeks or months after delivery (Gaynes et al. 2005). *Note*: 50% of "post-partum" major depressive episodes actually begin prior to delivery.

-9-

Compared to individuals with major depressive disorder, those with persistent depressive disorder (dysthymia) are at higher risk for which of the following comorbidities?

A. Bipolar disorder
B. Schizophrenia
C. Substance use disorders
D. Cluster A personality disorders
E. Posttraumatic stress disorder

Answer C: Compared to individuals with major depressive disorder, those with persistent depressive disorder (dysthymia) are at higher risk for psychiatric comorbidity, particularly anxiety and substance use disorders. Early-onset persistent depressive disorder is strongly associated with Cluster B and C personality disorders.

-10-
A 50-year-old man presents to outpatient clinic this morning complaining of mildly depressed mood. He has been
irritable, fatigued, experiencing headaches, temper outbursts, and having difficulty concentrating. He has never
felt down before and lately has been exercising and eating
healthier. Just yesterday he decided to eliminate sweets
from his diet and give up caffeinated beverages, as he is
a daily soda and coffee drinker. He drinks alcohol socially
and his last alcoholic beverage was 3 nights ago. Which
of the following explains his presenting symptoms?

A. Disruptive mood dysregulation disorder
B. Substance-Induced Depressive Disorder
C. Unspecified Depressive Disorder
D. Caffeine Withdrawal
E. Alcohol Withdrawal

Answer D: The patient's symptoms began within 24 hours
of cessation of caffeinated beverages. He is experiencing symptoms of caffeine withdrawal which can include:
headache, fatigue, dysphoric mood, difficulty concentrating, and flu-like symptoms.

-11-

Which of the following is the only non-substance-related addictive disorder recognized in the DSM-5 chapter on addictive disorders?

A. Gambling disorder
B. Internet gaming disorder
C. Social media addictive disorder
D. Compulsive computer gaming
E. Compulsive shopping

Answer A: No other excessive behavioral problems, including those associated with computer or Internet use, have sufficient research evidence to be included in this chapter. Internet gaming disorder has been included in the Appendix of DSM-5 to encourage further research.

-12-
Which of the following symptoms develop within several hours to a few days after cessation of alcohol to indicate alcohol withdrawal?

A. Nystagmus and incoordination
B. Dysphoric mood and rhinorrhea
C. Headache and flu-like symptoms
D. Irritability and decreased appetite
E. Insomnia and nausea/vomiting

Answer E: Insomnia and nausea/vomiting are alcohol withdrawal symptoms.   Nystagmus and incoordination are symptoms of alcohol intoxication. Headache and flu-like symptoms are typically present in caffeine withdrawal.   Dysphoric mood and rhinorrhea are usually seen in the opioid withdrawal. Irritability and decreased appetite are related to cannabis withdrawal.

-13-

A 21-year-old Caucasian man was recently diagnosed with paranoid schizophrenia. After a few doses of an atypical antipsychotic, he wakes up one morning confused, pale, and dysarthric. He is rigid throughout his extremities and warm to touch. His parents rush him to the ED for medical attention. Vital signs include: temperature 101°F, blood pressure 145/85, heart rate 112, and respiratory rate 22. Neuroleptic malignant syndrome (NMS) is highly suspected. Preliminary workup reveals leukocytosis, elevated creatine kinase and liver enzymes, and normal CT findings, consistent with NMS. Which of the following is also associated with this syndrome?

A. Metabolic alkalosis
B. Increased serum iron concentration
C. Generalized slowing on electroencephalography (EEG)
D. Agranulocytosis
E. Increased opening pressure on spinal tap

Answer C: Common abnormalities and laboratory findings in patients with NMS include: metabolic acidosis, hypoxia, leukocytosis (10,000 to 40,000/mm^3), elevated creatine kinase (1,000 to 10,000 IU/L), and mild elevations of: transaminases, alkaline phosphatase, and lactate dehydrogenase. Decreased serum iron concentration is also commonly seen and is a sensitive (but not specific) marker for NMS. Cerebrospinal fluid analysis and neuroimaging are generally normal. EEG can show generalized slowing.
[Source: http://www.uptodate.com/contents/neuroleptic-malignant-syndrome#H133036425]

-14-

A 72-year-old man with a history of hypertension and hyper-cholesterolemia presents to your clinic with his wife for an evaluation of memory problems. According to his wife, in the past few years after his stroke, he has become more forgetful of dates and family members' names. He gets confused more easily, often forgetting what he is doing and where he is going, leading to him wandering outside the house and being unable to drive. He also is unable to pay the bills anymore. Lately, after a hospitalization for a "mini stroke," he has been having difficulty speaking, described as "forgetting what things are called" and is having difficulty dressing and feeding himself. Which of the following is the most likely diagnosis?

A. Major Cognitive Disorder due to Alzheimer's Disease
B. Major Frontotemporal Neurocognitive Disorder
C. Major Vascular Neurocognitive Disorder
D. Major Neurocognitive Disorder with Lewy Bodies
E. Delirium

Answer C: Vascular neurocognitive disorder is charac-terized by neurocognitive symptoms temporally related to one or more cerebrovascular events. Decline is most prominent in complex attention and frontal-executive function.

-15-

A 70-year-old woman with a history of alcohol use disorder is day 10 of hospital admission from her assisted living facility for dehydration due to acute gallstone pancreatitis and protracted vomiting. After ERCP and removal of the gallstone in the common bile duct, she beings to improve and remains on parenteral intake due to continued vomiting and nausea. She remained in the hospital for vomiting but after it resolved she developed acute inattention and confusion 3 days ago. She is slightly better during the morning. On exam she is able to tell you her name but is disoriented to time and place. She has difficulty looking to the left and appears to be picking at something on her clothing. The rest of the exam is unremarkable. Her CT scan is negative for acute changes, including hemorrhage. Routine labs are normal as are amylase, lipase, lactate, and bilirubin levels. She is not able to focus to complete a MMSE. What is the most likely diagnosis?

A. Major Neurocognitive Disorder Due to Alzheimer's Disease
B. Major Vascular Neurocognitive Disorder
C. Alcohol withdrawal delirium
D. Delirium due to vitamin deficiency
E. None of the above

Answer D: Answer choices A and B can be eliminated, as the patient presents with an acute change in mental status. While she does have a significant history of alcohol abuse, she was in the hospital for 7 days with no alcohol intake prior to developing delirium. Delirium tremens tends to develop within 5 days of alcohol cessation. This patient has symptoms characteristic of Wernicke's encephalopathy, including ophthalmoplegia and confusion. She is at risk for undernourishment due to her continued vomiting and need for parenteral feeding which may not have adequately replenished her vitamin B1 stores. Thiamine supplementation is essential in preventing worsening cognition and memory problems.

-16-
Which one of the following neurocognitive disorders includes visual hallucinations and parkinsonism?

A. Neurocognitive disorder due to Prion disease
B. Neurocognitive disorder due to Huntington's disease
C. Neurocognitive disorder due to HIV infection
D. Neurocognitive disorder with Lewy Bodies
E. Frontotemporal neurocognitive disorder

Answer D: Visual hallucinations and parkinsonism are core diagnostic features of neurocognitive disorder with Lewy Bodies. Other features include fluctuation in cognition and attention, rapid eye movement sleep behavior disorder, and sensitivity to neuroleptics. Neurocognitive disorder due to prion disease is characterized by myoclonus and ataxia and confirmed by biopsy or autopsy. Frontotemporal neurocognitive disorder is characterized by behavioral and personality changes and/or language impairment.

-17-

A 48-year-old former football player, now private football coach, presents to your office accompanied by his wife. He reports coming to your office on his wife's insistence due concerns of his gradual decline in concentration over the past 3 years. He continues to work and remains independent. There are no personality changes noted by his wife. Family history is insignificant. There is no known history of traumatic brain injury. Medical workup performed 6 months ago, including bloodwork, chest x-ray, and CT head did not show any findings of significance to explain his symptoms. He scores a perfect 30 out of 30 on the MMSE performed in your office. He is referred for neuropsychiatric testing and the results come back showing that he is between 1-2 standard deviations below the mean in tests of complex attention while other areas of testing do not show any significant abnormalities. What is the most likely diagnosis?

A. Mild neurocognitive disorder due to Alzheimer's disease
B. Mild neurocognitive disorder
C. Major neurocognitive disorder
D. Mild neurocognitive disorder due to traumatic brain injury
E. Major neurocognitive disorder due to traumatic brain injury

Answer B: The neurocognitive disorders (NCD) can be classified as mild versus major. In major NCD there is significant cognitive decline, interference with independence, and the deficit(s) are not due to delirium or another mental disorder. In mild NCD there is mild to moderate cognitive decline and independence is not affected. Mild NCD was formerly classified as cognitive disorder NOS. Severity of the NCD can be determined with cognitive testing, though this alone should not be the main determinant of dysfunction and premorbid level of functioning must be taken into consideration. There is no known history of traumatic brain injury, though traumatic brain injury is much more common in football players. There is not enough information to support a diagnosis of Alzheimer's dementia.

-18-
Which of the following helps differentiate major neurocognitive disorder from mild neurocognitive disorder?

A. Concern of the individual
B. Impairment documented by neuropsychological testing
C. Interference with independence in everyday activities
D. Comorbid delirium
E. Comorbid psychiatric disorder

Answer C: While there is a modest amount of cognitive impairment in mild neurocognitive disorder, it does not interfere with independence in everyday activities, unlike the case with major neurocognitive disorder.

-19-

Which of the following is one of the six cognitive domains used to define the various neurocognitive disorders?

A. Language
B. Social cognition
C. Abstraction
D. Both A & B
E. Both A & C

Answer D: The six cognitive domains include: (1) complex attention, (2) executive function, (3) learning and memory, (4) language, (5) perceptual-motor, and (6) social cognition.

-20-
A 38-year-old meat factory worker is admitted to inpatient psychiatry for bizarre behavior. Neurology was consulted for newly developed ataxia and myoclonus. The patient becomes mute with major neurocognitive decline within days and is transferred to the neurology service. A few days later she dies in the intensive care unit. The patient was single with no children and did not have any major medical problems. What is the most likely diagnosis?

A. Major neurocognitive disorder due to prion disease
B. Major neurocognitive disorder due to HIV infection
C. Major neurocognitive disorder due to Parkinson's disease
D. Major neurocognitive disorder with Lewy bodies
E. Major neurocognitive disorder due to Huntington's disease

Answer A: Individuals with prion disease present with neurocognitive deficits, ataxia, and abnormal movements such as myoclonus, chorea, or dystonia; a startle reflex is also common. Typically, the history reveals rapid progression to major NCD in as little as 6 months.

-21-

A 70-year-old Caucasian man with no prior psychiatric history is admitted to the hospital for congestive heart failure and found to have severe aortic stenosis. Per nursing staff, he has been getting agitated, pulling out intravenous lines, and demanding to leave the hospital to walk his dogs. On evaluation, he is pleasantly smiling and appears to be in no acute painful or emotional distress. He is aware he is in the hospital, but thinks the year is 1956. Which of the following is a feature of delirium that can help differentiate it from dementia?

A. Memory loss
B. Inattention
C. Fluctuating course
D. Disorganized thinking
E. Agitation

Answer C: Fluctuating course is a diagnostic criterion for delirium. In the dementia syndromes, the course usually involves a steady or stepwise decline in functioning without return to baseline. Memory loss can be present in both delirium and dementia. Slow onset is characteristic of dementia, not delirium, which has an acute onset.

-22-

A 45-year-old woman presents to the emergency room with complaints of increased urinary frequency, headaches, backaches, lower abdominal pain, and numbness in her fingers for the past seven months. She reports that she has been missing deadlines at work due to appointments with different doctors and constantly worries about her health. She was informed by her doctor that all her basic labs, including abdominal ultrasound are within normal limits. What is the correct diagnosis?

A. Illness anxiety disorder
B. Somatic symptom disorder
C. Factitious disorder
D. Brief somatic symptom disorder
E. Malingering

Answer B: In somatic symptom disorder there are disproportionate thoughts about the seriousness of the symptoms and high levels of anxiety about the symptoms that are present. Symptoms are usually present for more than 6 months. Excessive energy and time are spent secondary to these health concerns. In illness anxiety disorder the patient is preoccupied about suffering from a serious illness. In factitious disorder, an individual presents as sick or impaired to others. In brief somatic symptom disorder, symptoms last less than six months.

-23-

A 26-year-old non-combat Iraqi War army veteran presents complaining of six month history of anxiety. He reports intense anxiety of being outside his home alone or in large crowds of people. He fears that escape in such situations may be difficult or that he will not be able to get help if he develops panic-like symptoms, such as palpitations or dizziness, which he experienced once before during a Fourth of July parade. He recognizes that his anxiety is excessive and he feels sad, because it has limited his social life. When asked about his military experiences, he mentions he witnessed several dead bodies in Afghanistan but does not endorse any re-experiencing symptoms, such as nightmares or flashbacks. He states he has moved on from his military experience and the discipline he gained while in active duty has helped him do well in his civilian IT job. He has a supportive wife and two young healthy children, ages three and five at home. He is a life-time nonsmoker, drinks rarely at social occasions, and denies illicit drug use now or ever in the past. What is his diagnosis?

A. Posttraumatic stress disorder (PTSD)
B. Panic disorder
C. Agoraphobia
D. Unspecified anxiety disorder
E. Separation anxiety disorder

Answer C: The patient suffers from agoraphobia, which is defined by DSM-5 as having marked fear or anxiety for 6 months or more about two or more of the following five situations: (1) using public transportation, (2) being in open spaces, (3) being in enclosed spaces, (4) standing in line or being in a crowd, or (5) being outside of the home alone. These situations are avoided because of thoughts that escape might be difficult or help might not be available in the event of developing panic-like symptoms or other incapacitating or embarrassing symptoms. The diagnosis of panic disorder requires the presence of recurrent, unexpected attacks. PTSD requires history of a traumatic life event along with re-experiencing, hyperarousal, numbing, avoidance, and negative alterations in cognitions and mood symptoms. While the patient does report irritability--a hyperarousal symptom in PTSD—he does not feel traumatized by his military experience, report nightmares/ flashbacks, or describe avoidance symptoms.

-24-

The criteria for posttraumatic stress disorder have changed in DSM-5. The previous three clusters were: re-experiencing, avoidance/numbing, and hyperarousal symptoms. In DSM-5, the avoidance cluster has been divided further into two distinct categories: avoidance and which of the following?

A. Problems with concentration
B. Sleep disturbance
C. Distressing dreams
D. Negative alterations in cognitions and mood
E. Hypervigilance

Answer D: The refined diagnostic criteria for posttraumatic stress disorder in DSM-5 splits the avoidance/numbing cluster into two categories: avoidance and negative alterations in cognitions and mood. This latter category requires that two or more of the following must be experienced and associated with the traumatic event: (1) inability to remember important aspects of the traumatic event, (2) persistent and exaggerated negative beliefs or expectations about oneself/others/world, (3) persistent and negative distortions about the cause or consequence of the event, (4) persistent negative emotional state, (5) markedly diminished interest in or participation in significant activities, (6) feelings of detachment from others, or (7) persistent inability to experience positive emotions. Problems with concentration, sleep disturbance, and hypervigilance (answer choices A, B, and E) are all hyperarousal symptoms found in the 'marked alterations in arousal and reactivity' cluster. Distressing dreams (answer choice **C**) are a part of the intrusion symptoms cluster.

-25-
A 24-year-old student presents to outpatient clinic complaining of intense "anxiety attacks," characterized by feeling extremely nervous and shaky, with sweaty palms. These symptoms occur when he is meeting new people for the first time, asking questions in class, or making oral presentations. Symptoms last until he is alone or in the company of close friends or family members. Symptoms occur when he has to talk in front of others and he is constantly worried about being embarrassed. Due to these symptoms for the past year, he avoids participating in class and going to parties with too many new faces. Which of the following is the most likely diagnosis?

A. Panic disorder with agoraphobia
B. Social anxiety disorder
C. Generalized anxiety disorder
D. Panic disorder without agoraphobia
E. Adjustment disorder

Answer B: Social anxiety disorder is defined as marked fear or anxiety about one or more social situations in which the individual is exposed to possible scrutiny by others. The individual fears that he or she will act in a way that will be negatively evaluated. The social situations almost always provoke fear and anxiety that is out of proportion to the threat. These situations are endured with intense fear or avoided and last at least 6 months or more.

NOTES

Test #2

-26-
A mother brings her 8-year-old son for evaluation. She explains for the past six months her child has been irritable, throwing tantrums, and seems to "freeze" while awaiting for the school bus, and "clings" to her when it arrives. She now finds herself driving him to and from school, as he has similar reactions while waiting for the bus to return home. The mother reports at home the child is comfortable and does not display any anxiety symptoms. Which of the following is the most likely diagnosis?

A. Separation Anxiety disorder
B. Specific phobia, situational type
C. Agoraphobia
D. Panic disorder
E. Panic attack

Answer B: The child has marked fear related to a specific situation (riding the school bus).

-27-

A 17-year-old high school student has been engaging in nightly binge-eating episodes for the past 4 months. She eats large quantities of fast food, such as 12 pieces of fried chicken, 3 orders of mashed potatoes, and 2 slices of pie in a 2 hour period while alone in her bedroom. Afterwards, she feels full and disgusted with herself. During the day, she watches her calories and has an adequate intake of food, but also uses laxatives and purges in the school bathroom. She constantly checks herself in the mirror to make sure she doesn't look fat. She wants to be thin and beautiful like the models she sees in fashion magazines. Her friends constantly reassure her that she looks fine—in fact, they tell her she is too thin. Her BMI is 15. What personality disorder is most closely associated with her eating disorder?

A. Borderline personality disorder
B. Obsessive compulsive personality disorder
C. Histrionic personality disorder
D. Narcissistic personality disorder
E. Avoidant personality disorder

Answer B: The student is excessively fearful of gaining weight and her inappropriate compensatory behaviors have resulted in an extremely low body weight. Her presentation meets criteria for anorexia nervosa, binge-eating/purging type. Although there is no weight criterion, patients with bulimia typically maintain normal body weight and those with binge-eating disorder are usually overweight. Anorexia is associated with obsessive-compulsive personality disorder, so answer choice B is correct here. *Note:* Other psychiatric diagnoses associated with anorexia include: major depression (65%), social phobia (34%), and obsessive-compulsive disorder (26%).

-28-
A 27-year-old respiratory therapist with no prior psychiatry history is admitted to the medical floor with intractable vomiting for the third time within the past six months. About a year prior to the onset of vomiting episodes, the patient was briefly hospitalized after a motor vehicle accident. The cause of vomiting has not been identified despite extensive diagnostic testing. The patient insists that there should be a medical reason behind her vomiting. Per nursing staff, the patient vomits much less than she reports. No evidence of external secondary gain to explain the patient's behavior can be identified. What is the most likely diagnosis?

A. Somatic symptom disorder
B. Malingering
C. Conversion disorder
D. Factitious disorder
E. Illness anxiety disorder

Answer D: The patient vomits much less than she reports but does not appear to have any external secondary gain from falsification of her symptoms. Her most likely diagnosis is factitious disorder. In somatic symptom disorder an individual has excessive attention- and treatment- seeking behavior for perceived medical concerns. In conversion disorder, neurological symptoms are reported without neurologic pathophysiology. In illness anxiety disorder, the individual is preoccupied by thoughts of having a serious disease in the absence of somatic symptoms, or if present, symptoms are only mild in intensity.

-29-

An 18-year-old woman is brought in by her mother because she has witnessed her eating toilet paper. The mother also reports her daughter has been vomiting frequently. On physical exam you observe a tall thin woman with a BMI of 17 kg/m², with no apparent physical abnormalities. On interview she eventually admits to consuming both tissues and toilet paper because they have no calories. She also admits she sometimes eats large amounts of food and then uses laxatives or purges to compensate for her behavior because she feels fat. What is the most likely diagnosis?

A. Pica
B. Anorexia nervosa
C. Binge eating disorder
D. Bulimia nervosa
E. Avoidant/restrictive food intake disorder

Answer B: The patient presents with low BMI, disturbance in body perception, and purging after binge-eating. When the ingestion of non-nutritive, non-food substances are primarily used as a means of weight control, anorexia nervosa is the primary diagnosis.

-30-

Which of the following criteria best differentiates bulimia nervosa from binge-eating disorder?

A. Sense of lack of control
B. Feelings of shame or guilt
C. Normal body weight
D. Recurrent inappropriate compensatory behavior
E. Frequent attempts at dieting

Answer: D. Bulimia nervosa and binge-eating disorder both have the criterion of recurrent episodes of binge-eating. Feelings of shame or guilt may accompany or follow the episodes in both disorders. Although individuals with both disorders may report frequent attempts at dieting, recurrent inappropriate compensatory behavior (e.g. purging, marked dietary restriction, driven exercise) is a criterion for bulimia nervosa but is an exclusion criterion for binge-eating disorder.

-31-

Which of the following is a key feature of factitious disorder?

A. Somatic symptoms
B. Misrepresentation of signs and symptoms
C. External gain associated with illness
D. Absence of another medical disorder that may cause the symptoms
E. Normal physical exam and laboratory tests

Answer B: The key feature of factitious disorder, whether imposed on oneself or on another, is the conscious and intentional reporting and misrepresentation of signs and symptoms of disease in order to receive medical attention, without other obvious external gain. A medical disorder associated with similar symptom presentation may be present, but if the patient knowingly misrepresents himself or herself, factitious disorder may be present.

-32-

Which of the following is correct regarding the diagnosis of intermittent explosive disorder?

A. Aggressive outbursts must be physical in nature
B. **Aggressive outbursts can be either physical or verbal in nature**
C. Chronological age must be at least 9 years
D. Destruction of property or physical injury must occur
E. Outbursts are committed to achieve a tangible objective, such as money, power, or intimidation

Answer B: DSM-5 now includes both verbal aggression and non-destructive/non-injurious physical aggression in the diagnostic criteria for intermittent explosive disorder. Chronological age must be at least 6 years, making answer choice C incorrect. The outbursts are neither premeditated nor committed for personal gain, making answer choice E incorrect.

-33-
A 52-year-old man eats at Old Country Buffet once a week. He eats more at the table than anyone else around him and seems to lack a sense of control over his excessive eating. He feels he deserves to eat what he wants after working long days on the farm. Despite his increasing girth, he feels his overeating is not problematic. His primary care physician educates him about the consequences of being overweight. He tells the doctor "I'll think about it" and appears to mean it. He decides to exercise 30 minutes on the weekends to lose weight. What is his most likely diagnosis?

A. Bulimia nervosa
B. Binge-eating disorder
C. Anorexia nervosa, binge-eating type
D. No DSM-5 diagnosis
E. Other specified feeding or eating disorder

Answer D: Though this man's eating habits can be considered unhealthy, his activities are not causing impairment at work or home. Also, the patient does not have preoccupation with his weight and has started a healthy exercise regimen to improve his weight. This patient does not meet criteria for an eating or feeding mental health disorder as defined by the DSM-5. He would be best helped by education on obesity, healthy eating patterns, and exercise encouragement, as provided by his primary care doctor. In defining disorders in the DSM-5, both (a) pathological patterns and (b) functional impairment and/or marked distress are necessary to diagnose someone with a mental illness.

-34-
A 30-year-old woman comes to clinic complaining of recurrent episodes of visual distortions, hypoemotionality, feeling robotic, and detached from her whole self. She is fearful of going crazy and having irreversible brain damage due to her symptoms. Which of the following is true about the disorder this woman most likely has?

A. Reality testing remains intact
B. There is high comorbidity with posttraumatic stress disorder
C. It commonly co-occurs with schizotypal personality disorder
D. It commonly occurs in women
E. It is usually caused by hallucinogens

Answer A: Reality testing remains intact in depersonalization/derealization disorder and is key to differentiating it from psychotic disorders. Lifetime comorbidities with depression and anxiety are high, while comorbidity with posttraumatic stress disorder is low. Avoidant, borderline, and obsessive-compulsive are the three most commonly co-occurring personality disorders. The male-to-female ratio is 1:1. Intoxication or withdrawal from illicit drugs such as marijuana, ketamine, ecstasy, hallucinogens, and salvia can cause depersonalization/derealization symptoms. However, an individual is not diagnosed with this disorder unless symptoms persist for some time in the absence of substance use.

-35-

A 22-year-old woman comes to your office complaining of multiple scab marks on her upper extremities and an unrelenting urge to pick her skin. She reports she feels less tense after picking her skin, and upon further interview it appears the skin picking is not in response to an obsession or done to prevent something bad from happening to her. She denies visual or tactile hallucinations, does not believe she has a rash or infection, and does not feel her arms are otherwise deformed. She denies alcohol or illicit drug use and has no medical problems. Due to her scabs, she has to take off from work and avoids going out socially. Which of the following is the most likely diagnosis?

A. Body dysmorphic disorder
B. Excoriation disorder
C. Obsessive compulsive disorder
D. Adjustment disorder
E. Generalized anxiety disorder

Answer B: Excoriation disorder involves skin picking that causes lesions and is difficult to control and/or stop. It is not due to a perceived defect, delusion, obsession, or compulsion. It causes significant impairment in daily functioning. It is not due to substance withdrawal or intoxication or medical problems.

-36-

A couple recently adopted a 4-year-old child from an orphanage in a war-stricken country. Very little is known about the child's history, except that she lost all her family at 2 months of age. She was found barely breathing in the rubble of a destroyed neighborhood. She was brought to a hospital, then to several shelters, and finally taken up by an orphanage in a small village quite far from where she was originally found. The adoptive parents are noticing that the child barely talks, has poor eye contact, appears sad and fearful for no reason, and has frequent unexplained episodes of irritability. She interacts poorly with the parents and other children. What is the most likely diagnosis?

A. Autism spectrum disorder
B. Intellectual developmental disorder
C. Major depressive episode
D. Reactive attachment disorder
E. Normal reaction to extreme stressors

Answer D: The patient has a history of severe social neglect and exhibits emotional dysregulation. She suffers from reactive attachment disorder. It can be difficult to differentiate from autism since both disorders involve delays in language development and problems with social interactions. Repetitive behaviors are, however, more common in autism. Children suffering from major depression may have impaired attachments, but often respond to comfort.

-37-

Personality disorders should NOT be diagnosed on the basis of problems associated with:

A. Interpersonal functioning
B. Affectivity
C. Cognition
D. Impulse Control
E. Acculturation following immigration

Answer E: The diagnosis of a general personality disorder requires an enduring pattern of behavior and inner experience in two of the following areas: cognition (ways of perceiving and interpreting self, other people, and events), affectivity (the range, intensity, lability, and appropriateness of emotional response), interpersonal functioning, and impulse control. Thus, answer choices A, B, C, and D are incorrect. The behavior of individuals with a personality disorder deviates markedly from the expectations of his or her own culture. However, the individual's ethnic, cultural, and social background must be taken well into account before making judgments about personality functioning. Problems associated with acculturation following immigration (answer choice E) or with the expression of habits, customs, religious values, and political values held by one's culture must not be confused as a personality disorder. Only when personality traits are inflexible, maladaptive, and cause significant personal impairment or subjective distress, do they represent a personality disorder.

-38-

A 21-year-old man presents to his primary medical doctor with his mother for an annual check-up. She reports wanting a second opinion for his "weird behavior." She reports that the patient has always been eccentric. She reports that he believes he has extra-sensory perception (ESP) and speaks as if he were a fortune-teller to family members. He has also has a tendency to wear odd combinations of patterns and has not made any friends while away at college. He has never complained of mood symptoms or auditory or visual hallucinations. Which of the following is the most likely diagnosis?

A. Schizophrenia
B. Schizophreniform Disorder
C. Schizoaffective Disorder
D. Schizotypal Personality Disorder
E. Schizoid Personality Disorder

Answer D: Schizotypal personality disorder is characterized by a pervasive pattern of interpersonal deficits marked by acute discomfort with, and reduced capacity for close relationships. Individuals with this personality disorder also have cognitive or perceptual distortions and eccentricities of behavior, beginning by early adulthood. These occur in a variety of contexts, as indicated by 5 or more of the following: ideas of reference, odd beliefs or magical thinking that influences behavior, unusual perceptual experiences, odd thinking and speech, suspiciousness or paranoid ideation, inappropriate or constricted affect, behavior or appearance that is odd, eccentric, or peculiar, lack of close friends, excessive social anxiety that does not diminish with familiarity.

-39-

Which of the following personality disorders is part of the schizophrenia spectrum of disorders?

A. Paranoid personality disorder
B. Schizoid personality disorder
C. **Schizotypal personality disorder**
D. Dependent personality disorder
E. Avoidant personality disorder

Answer C: Schizotypal personality disorder is characterized by odd beliefs or magical thinking, odd behavior or speech, lack of close relationships other than with relatives and ideas of reference that is pervasive, with a long enduring pattern of behavior that either causes distress or functional impairment. It may also be premorbid to schizophrenia. The symptoms of schizotypal personality disorder involve both positive symptoms such as ideas or reference and magical thinking and negative affect and decreased social behavior. Evidence has shown it is consistent with a disorder on the schizophrenia spectrum.

-40-
Why were subtypes of schizophrenia (i.e., paranoid, dis-organized, catatonic, undifferentiated, residual) removed from the DSM-5?

A. Poor validity
B. Low reliability
C. Limited diagnostic stability
D. A & B
E. All of the above

Answer D: The subtypes of schizophrenia (paranoid, disorganized, catatonic, undifferentiated, residual) were removed from DSM-V because they were found to have poor validity and low reliability. They also have limited diagnostic stability—they have not been shown to exhibit distinctive patterns with respect to longitudinal course. Furthermore, the subtypes were not found helpful in predicting treatment response or providing targeted treatment.

-41-

Which of the following is true concerning the onset of symptoms in attention-deficit/hyperactivity disorder (ADHD)?

A. Symptoms must cause impairment prior to age 7
B. **Inattentive or hyperactive-impulsive symptoms were present prior to age 12**
C. There is no age requirement for onset of symptoms as long as there is impairment at home and school
D. Inattentive symptoms occur more commonly in males
E. None of the above is true.

Answer B: The "B" criterion for ADHD, which describes the onset of symptoms, has been changed in DSM-5 to "several inattentive or hyperactive-impulsive symptoms were present prior to age 12." Previously, the criterion required "some hyperactive-impulsive or inattentive symptoms that caused impairment were present before age 7."

-42-

Which of the following is true regarding Tourette's Disorder?

A. The onset of symptoms must occur prior to age 12
B. Motor and vocal tics occur concurrently
C. Tics must persist for at least 2 years
D. **Both motor and vocal tics must occur at some time during the illness**
E. Either motor or vocal tics must occur during the illness

Answer D: For a diagnosis of Tourette's Disorder, both motor and one or more vocal tics must be present at some time during the illness prior to the age of 18, but are not required to occur concurrently. Symptoms can wax and wane but must persist for more than one year since the first tic occurs.

-43-

Childhood-onset fluency disorder involves problems with:

A. Sound and syllable repetitions
B. Social uses of verbal and nonverbal communication
C. Social-emotional reciprocity
D. Reduced vocabulary, including both word knowledge and use
E. Impaired ability to use vocabulary and explain a series of events

Answer A: Childhood-onset fluency disorder, or developmental stuttering, is a disturbance in the fluency of speech that is inappropriate for the individual's age. It is characterized by one or more of the following: sound and syllable repetitions, sound prolongations of consonants as well as vowels, broken words, audible or silent blocking, circumlocutions, words produced with an excess of physical tension, or monosyllabic whole-word repetitions.

-44-

Which of the following describes a condition or disorder which would be properly diagnosed as "Other Specified Sexual Dysfunction"?

A. Medical-induced sexual dysfunction
B. Sexual aversion
C. Erectile dysfunction
D. Female sexual interest/arousal disorder
E. Delayed ejaculation

Answer B: All of the answer choices except sexual aversion refer to diagnosable disorders in the sexual dysfunctions category, each with its own specific set of criteria. Sexual aversion, described as extreme aversion to and avoidance of genital sexual contact with a sexual partner, is given as an example of a presentation that is not currently recognized formally as a disorder. Sexual aversion would therefore be properly diagnosed as "Other Specified Sexual Dysfunction."

-45-
Which of the following is classified as an anxiety disorder?

A. Specific phobia
B. Obsessive-compulsive disorder
C. Selective mutism
D. Both A & B
E. Both A & C

Answer E: 'Obsessive-Compulsive and Related Disorders' is a new chapter in DSM-5, which includes hoarding disorder, excoriation (skin-picking) disorder, substance/medication-induced obsessive-compulsive and related disorder, and obsessive-compulsive and related disorder due to another medical condition. It is no longer characterized as an anxiety disorder.

-46-
The diagnosis of autism spectrum disorder includes all of the following, EXCEPT?

A. Deficits in social communication
B. Deficits in social interaction
C. Deficits in developing and maintaining relationships
D. Sound and syllable repetitions
E. Deficits in non-verbal communication behaviors

Answer D: Frequent repetitions or prolongations of sound and syllables are dysfluencies that occur in childhood-onset fluency disorder (stuttering). It is not one of the criteria for autism spectrum disorder.

-47-

For a diagnosis of hypersomnolence disorder, which of the following is true?

A. The hypersomnolence occurs at least two times per week, for at least two months
B. The hypersomnolence occurs at least five times per week, for at least one month
C. **The hypersomnolence occurs at least three times per week, for at least three months**
D. The hypersomnolence occurs for at least six months
E. The hypersomnolence occurs for at least one year

Answer C: Hypersomnolence is self-reported excessive sleepiness. The following symptoms are present in hyper-somnolence disorder: recurrent periods of sleep which occur within the same day or a prolonged sleep episode of more than nine hours within a day. These symptoms occur at least three times per week, for at least a three month period.

-48-

A 10-year-old girl with no past psychiatric history is brought for mental health evaluation after her mother noticed a change in her behavior for the past 7-8 months. The mother explains that the patient often loses her temper, has been vindictive at times, and recently confronted her school principal after she was suspended. Which of the following is the most accurate diagnosis?

A. Intermittent explosive disorder
B. Conduct disorder
C. Oppositional defiant disorder
D. Antisocial personality disorder
E. Borderline personality disorder

Answer C: Oppositional defiant disorder involves a pattern of angry/irritable mood, argumentative/defiant behavior or vindictiveness lasting at least 6 months with at least 4 of the following mood/behavior symptoms:
• Actively refuses to comply with majority's requests or consensus-supported rules
• Performs actions deliberately to annoy others
• Angry and resentful of others
• Argues often
• Blames others for his or her own mistakes
• Often loses temper
• Spiteful or seeks revenge
• Touchy or easily annoyed

Conduct disorder presents as repetitive and persistent pattern of behavior in which the basic rights of others or major age-appropriate norms are violated. Intermittent explosive disorder is a behavioral disorder characterized by extreme and impulsive expressions of anger, disproportionate to the situation at hand. To make a diagnosis of a personality disorder the individual must be at least 18 years old.

-49-

A 35-year-old man presents complaining of very poor sexual desire. He states that he has been having decreased interest in romantic relationships and sexual activity for over a year. He reports barely thinking about sex and not having the fantasies he used to have. Though he has never been much of a sexual creature he finds his nearly absent sexual desire problematic. He reports that he has been in a few relationships in the past and is currently single. He has stable employment, owns his house, and reports no medical problems. He does not smoke, drink or use any illicit drugs, and states that he is content professionally. What is the most likely diagnosis?

A. Major depressive disorder
B. Gender dysphoria
C. Unspecified sexual dysfunction
D. Male hypoactive sexual desire disorder
E. No psychiatric disorder

Answer D: This man does not meet criteria for major depression. There is also no evidence of gender dysphoria. The sexual dysfunction is related to the absence of sexual desire.

-50-

An 18-year-old man with no significant medical history presents to his primary care physician with complaints of excessive tiredness and daytime napping for the past 6 months. He is currently a freshman in college and is experiencing difficulty staying awake, especially during class. He notes that approximately 5-6 times per week he suddenly "collapses," associated at times with significant bruising. His BMI is 22 and routine labs reveal no abnormalities. Which of the following would the most appropriate next test to perform?

A. Magnetic resonance imaging of the brain
B. Lumbar puncture with cerebrospinal fluid analysis
C. Nerve conduction studies
D. Electroencephalogram
E. Urine toxicology

Answer B: This patient is most likely suffering from narcolepsy with cataplexy, which is characterized by recurrent periods of unrelenting desire to sleep for at least a three month period and at least three times per week, along with one of the following: (1) cataplexy (sudden bilateral loss of muscle tone with maintained consciousness triggered by emotions, such as laughing or crying), (2) hypocretin deficiency as measured using cerebrospinal fluid (CSF) hypocretin-1 immunoreactivity values, or (3) nocturnal sleep polysomnography showing rapid eye movement (REM) sleep latency less than or equal to 15 minutes, or other tests confirming the diagnosis. Lumbar puncture with CSF analysis would thus be the most appropriate next test to order.

NOTES

Test #3

-51-
A 28-year-old man with history of schizoaffective disorder presents to the emergency department after police find him agitated on the streets. He receives haloperidol 5mg intramuscularly 4 times in the course of 24 hours and is admitted to the inpatient psychiatric service. On day 2 of hospitalization he develops a painful twisting of his neck. Vital signs and laboratory tests are within normal limits. Which of the following is the most likely cause?

A. Medication-induced acute dystonia
B. Medication-induced akathisia
C. Tardive dyskinesia
D. Neuroleptic malignant syndrome
E. Medication-induced parkinsonism

Answer A: Medication-induced acute dystonia is characterized by abnormal and prolonged contraction of the muscles of the eyes, head, neck, limbs, or truck. Symptoms develop within a few days after starting, raising, or reducing the dosage of a medication used to treat extrapyramidal symptoms.

-52-

Which of the following is NOT considered to be one of the symptoms of caffeine intoxication?

A. Restlessness
B. Flushed Face
C. Rambling flow of speech
D. Periods of inexhaustibility
E. Headache

Answer E: Headache is a sign of caffeine withdrawal, not intoxication. Other signs of caffeine intoxication include: insomnia, increased urination, gastrointestinal discomfort, increased heart rate, arrhythmia, and psychomotor agitation.

-53-
A 17-year-old teenager is brought to the emergency department by his family. They report he is aggressive, confused, and producing nonsensical speech. His skin appears erythematous and dry; his pupils are dilated and he is noted to have involuntary eye movements. The family reports the patient had just returned from a party prior to presenting with above symptoms. What is the most likely diagnosis?

A. Cannabis intoxication
B. PCP intoxication
C. Alcohol intoxication
D. Caffeine withdrawal
E. Cocaine intoxication

Answer B: Signs and symptoms of PCP intoxication include: aggression, impulsive and unpredictable behaviors, vertical or horizontal nystagmus, hypertension or tachycardia, numbness, ataxia, dysarthria, muscle rigidity, seizures or coma, and hyperacusis.

-54-

A 19-year-old patient is brought to the emergency depart-ment by EMS for assaultive behavior. The patient states that he is "just fine," but refuses to change into a gown and is cursing and yelling at staff. He finally agrees to change and is examined by the resident psychiatrist. He is noted on mental status examination to have psychomotor retardation, slurred speech, and impaired judgment. Eye examination reveals nystagmus. Other positive findings include depressed reflexes and unsteady gait. The patient is most likely intoxication with which of the following?

A. PCP
B. Inhalant
C. Cocaine
D. Opioid
E. Cannabis

Answer B: Inhalant intoxication is characterized by behav-ioral changes, including belligerence, assaultiveness, and impaired judgment. Other findings include dizziness, nys-tagmus, slurred speech, unsteady gait, lethargy, depressed reflexes, psychomotor retardation, tremors, generalized muscle weakness, blurred vision, and euphoria. It is eas-ily confused with PCP intoxication, in which nystagmus and assaultive behavior are also present. However, other common findings include tachycardia, hyperacusis, and muscle rigidity. Nystagmus is not associated with opioid, cannabis, or cocaine intoxication.

-55-

Which of the following is true when differentiating mild or major neurocognitive disorder (NCD) with Lewy bodies from NCD due to Parkinson's disease?

A. In Parkinson's disease, cognitive decline occurs in the context of established Parkinson's disease; in NCD with Lewy bodies, cognitive symptoms occur before or concurrently with spontaneous parkinsonism
B. In Parkinson's disease, cognitive decline occurs before motor symptoms associated with Parkinson's disease; in NCD with Lewy bodies, cognitive symptoms occur after motor symptoms
C. Patients with Parkinson's disease are more likely to report visual hallucinations
D. NCD with Lewy bodies occurs more frequently in females
E. Parkinson's disease is a synucleinopathy due to alpha-synuclein misfolding and aggregation

Answer A: The timing of motor and cognitive symptoms helps distinguish between these two conditions. In Parkinson's disease, cognitive decline occurs at least one year after the motor and other associated symptoms of Parkinson's disease, i.e. the cognitive decline occurs in the context of established Parkinson's disease. In contrast, cognitive symptoms in NCD with Lewy bodies occur before or concurrently with spontaneous Parkinsonism. Both conditions occur more often in men; the male-to-female ratio is approximately 1.5:1 in Parkinson's disease. NCD with Lewy bodies, *not Parkinson's disease*, is a synucleinopathy due to alpha-synuclein misfolding and aggregation.

-56-

Which trinucleotide repeat is observed in the gene that encodes the huntingtin protein in Huntington's disease?

A. CAT
B. CAG
C. CAC
D. TAG
E. CCG

Answer B: Huntington's disease is an autosomal dominant disorder with complete penetrance. CAG is the trinueclotide repeat associated with this disease.

-57-

Loss of consciousness in mild traumatic brain injury (TBI) typically lasts for how long?

A. Less than 15 minutes
B. Less than 30 minutes
C. 30 minutes to 24 hours
D. Greater than 24 hours
E. Greater than 36 hours

Answer B: Severity ratings for traumatic brain injury are based on the following injury characteristics: (1) loss of consciousness, (2) posttraumatic amnesia, and (3) disorientation and confusion at initial assessment as per Glasgow Coma Scale Score. In mild TBI, these values are less than 30 minutes, less than 24 hours, and 13-15, respectively.

-58-

What is the most common cause of a traumatic brain injury (TBI)?

A. Falls
B. Motor vehicle accident
C. Sports concussions
D. Combat-related blasts
E. Gunshot wound

Answer A: The most common cause of TBI is falls followed by motor vehicle accident. Sports concussions are a common cause of TBI in adolescents and young adults.

-59-

An example of an assessment for sustained attention is:

A. Measuring time taken to put together a design of blocks
B. Hearing numbers and letters read and asking to count only numbers
C. Pressing a button every time a bell is heard
D. Rapidly tapping one's feet while carrying a conversation
E. Shifting from ordering objects by color to ordering by size

Answer C: Sustained attention is maintenance of attention over time. Pressing a button every time a bell is heard effectively assesses this. Answer choice A assesses processing speed, answer choice B assesses selective attention, answer choice D assesses divided attention, and answer choice E assesses cognitive flexibility.

-60-

Major risk factors for mild or major vascular neurocognitive disorder (NCD) include:

A. History of repeated falls
B. Thyroid dysfunction
C. Smoking
D. Low homocysteine levels
E. Sleep disorder

Answer C: Major risk factors for mild or major NCD include risk factors for cerebrovascular disease. This includes: diabetes, hypertension, hyperlipidemia, obesity, smoking, and high homocysteine levels. In addition, other conditions that increase the risk of cerebral emboli are also risk factors, such as atherosclerosis and atrial fibrillation.

-61-

Which of the following DOES NOT occur in delusional disorder?

A. More than one delusion
B. Bizarre delusions
C. Impaired functioning
D. Hallucinations
E. Brief major depressive episodes

Answer C: Delusional disorder is characterized by the presence of one or more delusions. The requirement that the delusions must be non-bizarre was removed from DSM-5, and a specifier for bizarre-type was added. Hallucinations may be present, as long as they are directly related to the delusion(s). People who have this disorder do not experience impairment in their daily functioning.

-62-

Obsessive-compulsive disorder (OCD) is characterized by:

A. Intrusive thoughts and repetitive behaviors
B. Either intrusive thoughts or repetitive behaviors
C. Excessive worrying
D. Guilty ruminations
E. Recurrent, pleasurable thoughts

Answer B: OCD is characterized by the presence of either obsessions (intrusive, unwanted thoughts) or compulsions (repetitive behaviors) that are time-consuming and cause distress or impairment in social, occupational, or other important areas of functioning.

-63-

Recurrent and intense sexual arousal from observing an unsuspecting person who is naked, in the process of disrobing, or engaging in sexual activity is:

A. Voyeuristic disorder
B. Exhibitionistic disorder
C. Frotteuristic disorder
D. Sexual sadism disorder
E. Fetishtic disorder

Answer A: Voyeuristic disorder is a paraphilic disorder in which the individual has acted on the aforementioned sexual urges with a nonconsenting person, or the sexual fantasies cause clinically significant distress or impairment in important areas of functioning.

-64-

What is the minimum length of time symptoms should be present for a diagnosis of delayed ejaculation?

A. 2 weeks
B. 6 weeks
C. 1-3 months
D. 6 months
E. 12 months

Answer D: Delayed ejaculation is defined as marked delay, infrequency, or absence of ejaculation on almost all occasions of partnered sexual activity (approximately 75%-100% of the time). Symptoms should be present for at least 6 months. Specifiers include: lifelong, acquired, generalized, or situational; severity of symptoms are rated as mild, moderate, or severe.

-65-

Alexithymia, a common occurrence in men diagnosed with psychogenic erectile dysfunction, is defined as:

A. Persistently low mood
B. Anxious affect
C. Intense emotional reactions
D. Affective blunting
E. Deficits in cognitive processing of emotions

Answer E: Deficits in cognitive processing of emotions is better known as alexithymia.

-66-
Taiijin kyofusho is:

A. "Interpersonal fear disorder"
B. "Fright"
C. "Weakness of the nervous system"
D. "Thinking too much"
E. "Wind attacks"

Answer A: In Taijin kyofusho, individuals feel their appearance or actions in social situations are inadequate to others, resulting in avoidance and anxiety about social situations. Susto is an illness attributed to a frightening event that causes the soul to leave the body and results in unhappiness and sickness, or "fright." Shenjing shuairuo is "weakness of the nervous system" and is defined as a syndrome composed of three out of five symptom clusters: weakness, emotions, excitement, nervous, and sleep. Kufungisisa, or "thinking too much," is an expression describing the distress that is considered to be causative of depression, anxiety, and somatic problems. Khyâl cap, or "wind attacks" refers to panic symptoms and is a syndrome found among Cambodian people.

-67-

How are illness anxiety disorder and somatic symptom disorder similar?

A. High levels of anxiety about health are experienced
B. Significant somatic symptoms are present
C. The individual performs excessive health-related behaviors
D. A & B
E. A & C

Answer E: In both disorders, there are high levels of anxiety and excessive health-related behaviors. However, somatic symptoms are minimal, if not absent, in individuals with illness anxiety disorder who are more concerned about being ill in general.

-68-

Disorders most commonly comorbid with pica are:

A. Autism spectrum disorder
B. Intellectual disability
C. Obsessive-compulsive disorder
D. A & B
E. A & C

Answer D: Patients who suffer from pica engage in the persistent eating of nonnutritive, nonfood substances for a period of at least one month. Autism spectrum disorder and intellectual disability are most commonly comorbid with pica.

-69-
Rumination disorder is:

A. Repeated regurgitation of food; the food is either re-chewed, re-swallowed, or spit out
B. Excessive attention to one's own distress in the setting of depressive symptoms
C. Characterized by recurrent, unwanted intrusive thoughts
D. Characterized by excessive time spent before making decisions commonly in the setting of a perfectionistic personality style
E. Related to excessive anxiety over making decisions related to everyday matters

Answer A: The repeated regurgitation of food occurring after feeding or eating over a period of at least one month is the main feature of rumination disorder.

-70-
Avoidant/restrictive food intake disorder is:

A. Avoidance of food based on the sensory characteristics of food
B. Avoidance of eating food in social situations secondary to anxiety about embarrassing oneself in public
C. Can be related to dependence on enteral feeding or oral Nutritional supplements
D. A & B
E. A & C

Answer E: Avoidant/restrictive food intake disorder is a feeding disturbance which can be characterized by: (1) lack of interest on feeding activity, (2) avoidance of food based on sensory characteristics of food, (3) concern about aversive consequences of eating. Associated features can include significant weight loss, nutritional deficiency, dependence on enteral feeding or oral nutritional supplements, or interference with social functioning.

-71-
Which of the following is true about dissociative amnesia?

A. Non-epileptic seizures may accompany dissociative amnesia
B. Is irreversible because neurobiological damage prevents memory storage and retrieval
C. Individuals with dissociative amnesia are frequently unaware of their memory problems
D. A & B
E. A & C

Answer E: Dissociative amnesia is characterized by an inability to recall important autobiographical information and often a lack of awareness of memory problems. This disorder can be further categorized as either: localized, generalized, systematized, or continuous. The amnesia is potentially reversible because the memories are successfully stored. Non-epileptic and other functional neurological symptoms may accompany dissociative amnesia.

-72-
Encopresis is:

A. Repeated voiding of urine into bed or clothes
B. Not diagnosed until a child has reached a chronological of at least 6 years
C. More common in females
D. **Often comorbid with urinary tract infections**
E. Most often intentional

Answer D: Encopresis is the repeated passage of feces into inappropriate places, usually done involuntarily but occasionally is intentional. It is not diagnosed until at least 4 years of age; approximately 1% of 5-year-olds have encopresis and it is more common in males. Encopresis can be comorbid with urinary tract infections, but this occurs more commonly in females.

-73-
What is the core feature of gender dysphoria?

A. Marked incongruence between one's experienced/ expressed gender and assigned gender
B. A strong preference for playmates of the other gender
C. A strong dislike of one's sexual anatomy
D. A strong preference for cross-gender roles
E. A strong desire for the sexual characteristics that match one's experienced gender

Answer A: Marked incongruence between one's experienced/expressed gender and assigned gender is the core component in the diagnosis of gender dysphoria. The other answer choices are associated criteria that can also be present in this disorder.

-74-
The prevalence of which of the following is higher in children with enuresis than in children without enuresis:

A. Autism spectrum disorder
B. Behavioral symptoms
C. Anxiety disorders
D. Tourette's disorder
E. Attention-deficit/hyperactivity disorders

Answer B: There is a higher prevalence of behavioral symptoms in children with enuresis. Developmental delays are present in a portion of children with enuresis. Sleepwalking and sleep terror can also be present. Most children with enuresis, however, do not have a comorbid mental disorder.

-75-

Which of the following is an example of a phase of life problem?

A. Bullying or intimidation by another individual
B. Retiring
C. Getting married
D. B & C
E. All of the above

Answer D: Examples of a phase of life problem include: beginning or completing school, leaving parental control, getting married, starting a new career, becoming a parent, adjusting to life after children leave home, and retiring. Bullying, teasing, and intimidation by others are examples of social exclusion or rejection.

NOTES

Part III

Directory

DSM-5 DIAGNOSTIC CATEGORIES AND CORRESPONDING QUESTIONS

1. Neurodevelopmental Disorders: 41, 42, 43, 46
2. Schizophrenia Spectrum and Other
    Psychotic Disorders: 40, 61
3. Bipolar and Related Disorders: 1, 2, 3, 4, 5
4. Depressive Disorders: 6, 7, 8, 9
5. Anxiety Disorders: 23, 25, 26, 45, 66
6. Obsessive-Compulsive and Related
    Disorders: 35, 62
7. Trauma- and Stressor- Related
    Disorders: 24, 36
8. Dissociative Disorders: 34, 71
9. Somatic Symptom and Related
    Disorders: 22, 28, 29,
                                     30, 31, 67
10. Feeding and Eating Disorders: 27, 33, 68, 69, 70
11. Elimination Disorders: 72, 74
12. Sleep-Wake Disorders: 47, 50
13. Sexual Dysfunctions: 44, 49, 64, 65
14. Gender Dysphoria: 73
15. Disruptive, Impulse-Control, and
    Conduct Disorders: 32, 48
16. Substance-Related and Addictive
    Disorders: 10, 11, 12,
                                     52, 53, 54
17. Neurocognitive Disorders: 14, 15, 16, 17,
                                     18, 19, 20, 21,
                                     55, 56, 57, 58,
                                     59, 60
18. Personality Disorders: 37, 38, 39
19. Paraphilic Disorders: 63

Mastering the New Psychiatric Diagnoses was written by the 2013-2014 residents and fellows of the Department of Psychiatry, Rutgers New Jersey Medical School, and then edited by Samina S. Raja, MD, and Petros Levouinis, MD, MA.

Samina S. Raja, MD, is a senior psychiatry resident at Rutgers New Jersey Medical School. She will continue her training as a fellow in geriatric psychiatry at Duke University, where she has been accepted for the next school year.

Petros Levounis, MD, MA, is the chair of the Department of Psychiatry at Rutgers New Jersey Medical School. He is a recipient of the National Institute of Mental Health Outstanding Resident Award, earned during the Columbia University residency-training program. He went on to complete a fellowship in addiction psychiatry at New York University, and is now a distinguished fellow of the American Psychiatric Association.